Doctor Guide Book Series
The Doctor's Guide to:

TREATING ALLERGIES

By
V.M. Taylor Hon.B.A., M.Sc.
Medical writer
In consultation with Dr. Philip Lieberman

Our thanks for being allowed to adapt educational material from the American Academy of Allergy Asthma & Immunology; the American College of Allergy, Asthma and Immunology; the Allergy Asthma Information Association, the American Pharmacists Association, the Canadian Pharmacists Association and the Physicians Association for Patient Education as well as the many physicians who provided their own educational material and provided editing and direction for the content.

The publisher acknowledges the financial support of the government of Canada through the Book Publishing Industry development Program (BPIDP) for our publishing activities.

Important disclaimer: Although all information in this book has been validated by authoritative professional bodies such as dosage regimens, the book is not intended to replace instructions from a health care professional.

ISBN # 978-1-896616-07-0

Printed in Canada

HOW TO:
Order More Copies of This Book

Tel: 800 773 5088,
Fax: 800 639 3186,
Email: **mediscript30@yahoo.ca**

Other Books in Our Allergy Series Include:

- Your Allergy-Free Home
- COPD Prevention and Treatment
- How to Stop Smoking
- Preventing Asthma Attacks
- Life - Threatening Anaphylaxis
- Allergy Avoidance in the Home

**For more information, visit us
at www.mediscript.net**

Foreword

Rhinitis, which is roughly translated as inflammation or 'disease of the nose', is arguably the most common human affliction.

In fact, all of us, at least periodically during our lives, suffer from rhinitis. This is because we all catch "the common cold". Recall the symptoms of the common cold and you will understand the illness first hand, for the symptoms of rhinitis are always the same, regardless of the cause.

They consist of those which we are all familiar, including runny nose, drainage down the back of the throat, stuffy and stopped up nose, sneezing and sometimes itching of the nose. These rhinitis symptoms are also classic allergy symptoms and often an allergy is known as "allergic rhinitis". People who have rhinitis constantly for weeks or months have chronic rhinitis..

Unfortunately since chronic rhinitis is a non fatal illness, it often gets little respect from those who do not have it, and even some physicians who care for patients with it. It has therefore been called "the Rodney Dangerfield of illnesses".

Personally, being a sufferer from chronic rhinitis (a fact which in part prompted my interest in becoming an allergist – immunologist) I am delighted to see that there is now a concise well written text "Treating Your Allergies" that deals with the problems posed by chronic rhinitis.

This easy reading text, written for the sufferer, is of great value because the informed patient, armed with knowledge of the illness and treatments, clearly suffers less.

This volume clearly transmits the type of information that we as allergists try to give our patients on a daily basis, but because of time limitations are not always successful in doing so.

This book will serve as a welcome supplement to our administrations, and is therefore an extremely useful tool for any patients suffering with the disorder.

Philip Lieberman MD

3

Contents

HOW TO USE THIS BOOK

You may have been given this book by a health care professional such as a physician or pharmacist because it takes a lot of time to explain how you manage an allergy condition.

You may be an allergy sufferer who takes non prescription medication for allergy symptoms and you are seeking as much information as possible to cope with the condition. This book will help you gain a comprehensive understanding.

The content of this book focuses upon only Allergic or non allergic Rhinitis which encompasses probably 95% of all allergies. Other allergies like skin allergies, severe allergic reactions (anaphylaxis), eye allergies (allergic conjunctivitis) and others are not covered.

As there is a lot of self medication taking place for allergies and there are also many people suffering from allergies who do not know they have allergies , this book could act as a catalyst to provide both understanding and with advice from your physician or pharmacist, the right treatment.

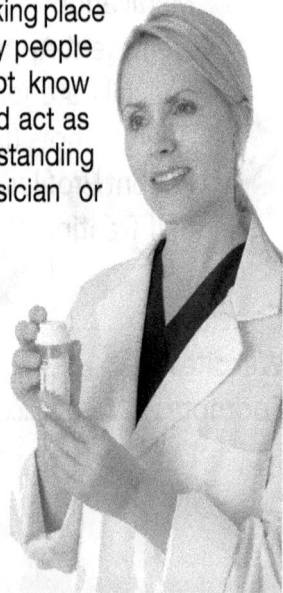

Tya032009c

INTRODUCTION

Allergic rhinitis is the most common form of allergies. Rhinitis relates to all the symptoms of the mucous membranes of the nose associated such as sneezing, itching, and runny nose.

More than 20% of adults and up to 40% of children suffer from allergic rhinitis, (the most common form of allergies), the intermittent or persistent symptoms include sneezing, runny nose, nasal conges-tion, watery eyes, and itching (pruritus). The prevalence continues to grow for unknown reasons

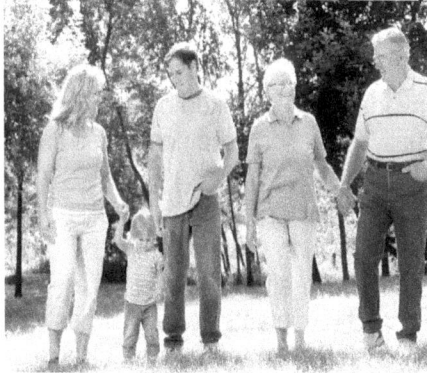

Traditionally allergic rhinitis has been divided into seasonal (hayfever) and perennial (lasting all year). However because an increasing number of patients are sensitized to both in-door and outdoor causes (allergens), the distinctions between these categories have become more blurred. An alternative classification has been proposed that classifies allergic rhini-tis on the basis of duration and severity of the symptoms. Health care professionals tend to now use a stepwise ap-proach to treatment with the choice of medication dictated by the symptoms.

The causes of allergies seem innocuous enough, such as mold spores, house dust mites, animal dander, pollen (from trees, grasses or weeds) and cockroaches. However the North American population seems to spend more and more time indoors so it is no surprise that these allergens or causes have become a health concern. In fact it has been reported in two studies that North Americans spend 90% of their time indoors and 20 hours of the day inside a building or home.

There are strict medical definitions of allergies but put simply, allergies are a misguided response by the body's immune system to normally harmless substances (allergens) like pollen or house dust mite. In allergic people, for reasons that are not entirely clear, these substances are viewed as potential invaders and attacked by the immune system. This attack actually turns upon the nose itself and causes the symptoms.

The causes mentioned above – pollen, house dust, mites and so on – bring on symptoms by being inhaled, but there are other ways allergens can enter your body: by way of skin contact e.g. plants, jewelry, ingested e.g. food and drugs and parenteral (penetrating the skin) e.g. insect stings or injections.

Your body's immune system is a protection mechanism designed to defend you against bacteria, viruses, parasites etc. and usually does a remarkable job. However, with allergies, the immune response is misdirected. Harmless substances look like invaders to the allergy patient. The good news though is that for the most part, allergies are not life threatening, apart from one serious allergic reaction "anaphylaxis" which will be discussed later. Allergies are mostly a debilitating quality of life issue which cannot be cured but the symptoms can usually be controlled.

The economic and health ramifications of allergic rhinitis are far reaching, more than 3.5 million work days and 2 million missed school days per year have been reported.

Allergic rhinitis is also associated with decreased on – the – job worker productivity or "presenteeism." When the costs caused by this "presenteeism" are calculated, employers pay a higher cost for allergic rhinitis than they do for asthma, cancer, diabetes or migraine.

It is estimated the medical costs can range from $2 – $ 5 billion. There are also more than 18 million physician office visits each year related to allergic rhinitis.

Further, allergic rhinitis may be associated with the development of other diseases such as asthma, rhinosinsusitis, otitis media and allergic conjunctivitis. Rhinitis can worsen asthma and predispose of it. This can occur in rhinitis due to allergy or other causes.

Allergic rhinitis has tended to be regarded as more of a nuisance than a condition that dictates repeat medical office visits. This traditional view, however, overlooks the profound impact that allergic rhinitis can have on a patient's quality of life, affecting both emotional well-being and everyday functioning. About half of all patients have symptoms for more than 4 months each year, while 20% of patients have symptoms for more than 9 months. In one study, 44% of patients with allergic rhinitis reported fatigue on awakening despite a normal night of sleep.

In light of this "nuisance" attitude towards allergic rhinitis, self management is very common. In the 2006 "Allergies in America" study – a telephone survey of 2,500 adults who had been diagnosed with allergic rhinitis and had experienced symptoms within the past 12 months – only 47% or respondents had seen a primary care physician about their nasal allergies during the past year. Of the patients who reported having used a medication for allergy symptoms during the past 4 weeks, the largest percentage (53%) had used a non prescription medication.

More worrying, self treatment with nonprescription medications also is believed to be common among the many people who experience symptoms consistent with allergic rhinitis, yet remain undiagnosed. These people often do not consider their symptoms to be "out of the ordinary" and thus see no need to consult with a medical provider.,

It has been estimated that as few as 12% of patients with rhinitis visit their physicians for treatment.

Apart from all the previous alarming statistics, the good news is that allergy symptoms can be controlled, prevented or minimized.

If you can find out what triggers your allergies and understand how to treat the disease, you can enjoy a normal productive, healthy lifestyle.

Managing your allergies consists of:

1. Avoid or minimize your exposure to the allergens (triggers/causes) and irritants through environmental control.

2. Use appropriate medication.

3. Immunotherapy (allergy shots) - taking a series of allergy

shots (injections) to de-sensitize against the allergen, similar in outcome to vaccinations.

4. Empower yourself through educating yourself and family members/caregivers on treatment issues and understanding the disease.

The components of actual medical treatment for allergies are shown in the "pie" below, even though we know some people just visit their pharmacies for advice and medication relief.

POSSIBLE TREATMENT STAGES FOR ALLERGIES

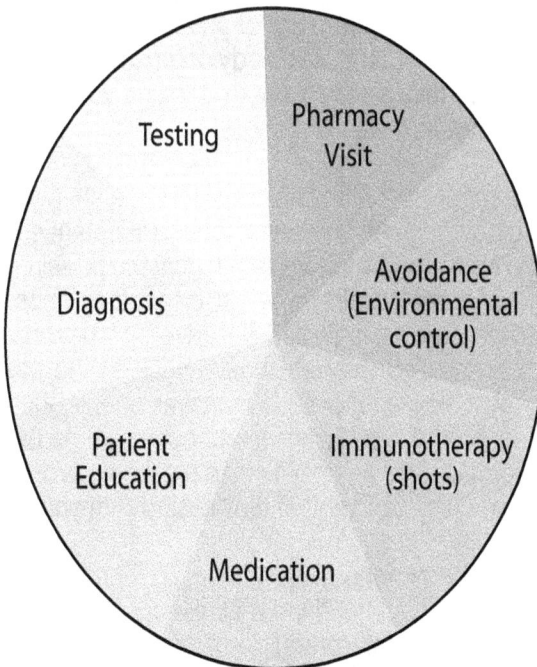

Testing

Pharmacy Visit

Diagnosis

Avoidance (Environmental control)

Patient Education

Immunotherapy (shots)

Medication

DIAGNOSIS

Causes of Allergies

When your nose is runny and your eyes are itchy you are probably just interested in relief, not in the causes of the symptoms or why this is happening. However, when you have a medical condition that you are likely to have for the rest of your life it can be helpful to understand what is going on so that you can cope with confidence.

We have already highlighted that the body's immune system is your main protective biochemical system to maintain health. Consider what happens to a human body when it dies – the immune system shuts down and in a matter of hours the body is invaded by all sorts of bacteria, microbes and the like that start to dismantle the body completely within weeks. None of these things were able to damage your body when the immune system was working.

A major component of the immune system is the lymphocyte (a white blood cell). As soon as a foreign substance (protein) enters the body, the lymphocytes identify the protein – fingerprinting it and determining whether or not it belongs. These lymphocytes can be regarded as traveling custom agents. Everywhere they go they are busy checking the passports of every cell they encounter. Whenever one of these cells poses danger to the body, the lymphocytes immediately begin countermeasures against it and a biochemical destructive action takes place to maintain the "security" of your body.

In allergies, the lymphocytes misidentify harmless proteins such as pollen or animal dander as serious enemies and react because of misinterpretation of the threat, causing the allergy symptoms to develop.

The lymphocyte, due to misguided response, instructs one of its cohorts, a second form of lymphocyte, to change into a cell called a plasma cell. It further instructs this plasma cell to manufacture an antibody called IgE, which is an immunoglobulin. All immunoglobulins are synthesized to fight invaders such as certain parasites. However for reasons unknown in the allergic population, the IgE is syntesized to fight the harmless substances, allergens, as previously noted. . This process is a sensitization phase which means on first exposure patients become sensitized and produce the IgE antibody.

Once the IgE antibody is produced, it circulates through the blood stream and binds to the cells called mast cells and basophils which both contain chemicals needed by the body to kill the parasites. These cells therefore are packages of potentially toxic chemicals such as histamine and leukotrienes. When IgE is used to kill parasites, these toxic chemicals are released to kill the parasites, but in allergic patient, upon re-exposure to allergen, these chemicals "attack the allergen". However they actually have no effect on these allergens. Unfortunately they do affect the nose.

Histamine is one of the most important of these chemicals. In the nose, it causes the glands to make mucus, the blood vessels to swell, producing nasal congestion and obstruction, the nerves to itch and cause sneezing, and can therefore produce all the symptoms noted above.

If you are an allergy sufferer you have probably heard of medications called antihistamines. They are called antihistamines because they are specifically designed to reverse the effects of histamine. Examples of such medications are those available are those that are available by prescription only are

Clarinex® (Aerius® in Canada), Allegra®, and Xyzal®, and those which one can purchase over – the - counter including Claritin®, Zyrtec® (Reactine in Canada), and Alavert®

Histamine, and other chemicals released from Mast cells and basophils, can exert reactions all through the body as well. These reactions depend on the site where histamine and other chemicals are present. The following chart shows the effect of these chemicals in other areas of the body, and the disease names used refer to these effects.

EFFECT OF HISTAMINE & OTHER CHEMICALS ON VARIOUS PARTS OF THE BODY

Allergic Disease/ Reaction	Site	Signs/symptoms
Rhinitis	Nose	Sneezing, rhinorrhea (runny nose), nasal itching, congestion
Asthma	Lungs	Coughing, wheezing, shortness of breath
Dermatitis	Skin	Itching, rash
Conjunctivitis	Eye	Itching, redness, tearing
Anaphyalxis	Systemic (all over the body)	Low blood pressure, shock, potential death
Food Allergy	Gut	Bloating, vomiting, diarrhea, cramping

We have explained how the body reacts abnormally to the usually harmless substances that you breathe in but let us now look at the complete list of the triggers that can cause the allergy problem (allergic rhinitis). Some substances in the list are not allergens. These substances are irritants. They do not act through the immune system, and problems that they cause are not truly allergies. They are not mediated by the actions of IgE, mast cells and basophils.

These substances include strong smells, respiratory irritants, and sometimes weather conditions such as changes in temperature and humidity, and 'a front coming in'. In addition true invaders, such as viruses, that cause common colds (viral respiratory tract infections) can also trigger symptoms similar to allergic rhinitis. However they are classified as non allergenic rhinitis, even though there are similar symptoms.

The most common form of non allergenic rhinitis is vasomotor rhinitis or VMR which can caused by a wide variety of irritants such as perfumes, strong smells, as mentioned previously. If you just have VMR you may only need a nasal spray and not an oral medication to treat this condition.

It is possible to have both VMR and allergic rhinitis, this is called mixed rhinitis.

Triggers or Causes of Your Rhinitis Symptoms

- Pollens from grass, trees and weeds
- Animal dander
- Cockroaches
- Irritants such as perfumes, odors, sprays, fumes
- House dust mites
- Molds / fungi
- Viral respiratory infections
- Tobacco smoke/Woodsmoke

Genetic causes (Atopy)

Atopy is another term for allergy. Allergies are inherited. People who have allergies are called atopic individuals. The term atopy in Greek refers to 'a strange place', meaning allergies were initially thought to be a rare and strange condition. Now allergies have become so prevalent that they are certainly no longer strange. Nonetheless the term atopy has persisited in the literature, and simply is a synonym for allergies.

Atopic conditions often occur together. For example, some people have a mixture of atopic skin disease (atopic dermatitis), rhinitis, and asthma.

The statistics show that 50% of atopic dermatitis patients develop asthma, and approximately 75% of atopic dermatitis patients develop allergic rhinitis.

The prevalence of atopic dermatitis in children is increasing; it is estimated that 10-15% of the population are affected by atopic dermatitis during childhood.

Drug induced rhinitis

Some medications can bring on rhinitis symptoms so it is important to know which drugs do this such as:

•Adrenergic antagonists,Angiotensin – converting enzyme inhibitors, •Aspirin and non steroidal anti inflammatories, •Chlorpromazine, •Intraocular preparations (e.g. B-Blockers), •Oral contraceptives, •Prozosin, •Adrenergic anatrogonists such as certain eye drops (containing beta-blocks) • Some anti-hypertensive medications • Aspirin and other nonsteroidal anti inflamtory drugs,

DO YOU HAVE AN ALLERGY?

Allergies are considered mostly in the category of a respiratory disease – as you probably know, there are lots of respiratory conditions such as asthma, colds, flu, sinusitis, and bronchitis.

As well as respiratory problems, allergies can also be in the category of skin disorders: eczema, atopic dermatitis and urticaria, for instance. To complicate matters further, there may be conditions that have an allergic component contributing to the problem: otitis media, conjunctivitis of the eye, food and drug reactions and insect sting reactions.

Anaphylaxis, a severe allergic reaction, is rare, although extremely serious and is most often caused by a reaction to drugs, certain foods or insect stings or bites. The nature of this allergic reaction is such that it affects all of the body; the drop in blood pressure and breathing problems that can occur make this condition life-threatening in a short period of time. An immediate injection of epinephrine (adrenaline) will relieve the condition; if you are at risk of anaphylaxis you should carry this injection with you at all times. The injection is easy to work and relatively painless and it is a life saver. The two brands that are available in North America are Epipen® and TwinJect®.

The biggest problem in diagnosing whether you have an actual allergy is in differentiating between other disorders such as flu, colds, sinusitis, and bronchitis.

As a general rule, allergic rhinitis can be differentiated from other respiratory disorders by the presence of sneezing, rhinorrhea (runny nose), nasal itching, and ocular symptoms such as itchy, watery, or red eyes. The table on the next page shows this:

18

SYMPTOMS COMMON FOR ALLERGIC RHINITIS

A. Watery, runny nose ☐

B. Sudden Sneezing ☐

C. Stopped up, or blocked nose ☐

D. Itching of nose ☐

E. Itching & redness of the eyes ☐

F. Occasional loss of smell ☐

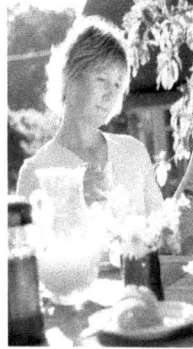

Generally speaking, allergic rhinitis symptoms are more intense during the morning in approximately 70% of patients. The symptoms tend to improve during the day and then worsen again in the evening. In addition to the characteristic symptoms, patients may experience diminished sense of smell and ability to taste, particularly if they have chronic, severe nasal congestion.

It is worth mentioning that allergic rhinitis may be associated with a number of complications and other diseases. These include asthma, sinusitis, nasal polyposis, lower respiratory tract infection and dental malocclusion.

On the following page all possible symptoms are listed, related to the three major respiratory problems of colds, allergic rhinitis and asthma. Place a tick on the symptom and match up your symptoms with the possible condition.

It must be emphasized the following chart is meant for information purposes only which may suggest the nature of your problem. You should consult your physician or pharmacist before taking any action.

Check Out Your Symtoms

SYMPTOM:	TICK IF YES:	ALLERGIES:	COMMON COLD:	ASTHMA:
Aches or pains	☐	Never	Common	Never
Chest Tightness	☐	Never	Rarely	Sometimes
Cough	☐	Sometimes	Common	Sometimes
Eyes - Skin just below is blue shade & swollen	☐	Common	Sometimes	Never
Fever	☐	Never	Occasionally	Never
Itchy watery or red eyes	☐	Common	Rare	Never
Itchy nose	☐	Common	Sometimes	Never
Itchy throat / mouth	☐	Common	Common	Never
Nasal congestion	☐	Common	Common	Never
Nasal discharge: thin, clear	☐	Common	Common	Never
Nasal discharge: thick, yellow	☐	Never	Common	Never
Postnasal drip	☐	Common	Common	Never
Runny nose	☐	Common	Common	Never
Shortness of breath	☐	Never	Never	Common
Sneezing all the time	☐	Common	Common	Never

TYPES OF RHINITIS

It is important to be familiar with the terminologies used to refer to the forms of rhinitis.

Rhinitis: an inflammation of the mucous membrane of the nose.

Allergic rhinitis: caused by IgE-mediated reactions of the nasal mucosa to one or more allergens such as pollen, food, or house dust.

Seasonal allergic rhinitis (also known as hayfever): like allergic rhinitis, but caused by one or more seasonal airborne allergen such as pollen.

Perennial allergic rhinitis: symptoms have no seasonal variation and are continuous throughout the year, usually caused by house dust mites, mold, cockroaches, animal dander or other airborne particles.

Non allergic rhinitis:

Vasomotor rhinitis: symptoms caused by non specific factors such as chemical irritants, strong smells, and climate changes.

Cholinergic rhinitis: defined by the excessive runny nose brought on by spicy foods or the inhalation of cold, dry air.

Infectious rhinitis: usually caused by a virus.

Rhinitis medicamentosa: caused by drugs such as overuse of nasal decongestant.

TESTING FOR ALLERGIES

Obviously, there are symptoms we associate with allergies, such as sneezing, runny nose, and watery eyes. The physician recognizes these symptoms as the first clues to a diagnosis of allergy. However, it must be emphasized that other medical problems can cause these same symptoms. This is why it is vitally important to visit your physician to ensure a correct diagnosis, so that you can get effective treatment.

Once the doctor knows your symptoms, he or she will ask a lot of questions to find out the "when, where, how, and what" of the allergy. If you suddenly start developing watery eyes and sneezing on the arrival of a kitten for your daughter, it is likely that you have developed an allergy to cat dander.

Many physicians have their own questionnaire for their patients to complete, so that they can systematically evaluate all of the possibilities. That, together with subsequent analysis of symptoms, will enable your physician to put forward some suggestions as to what is causing your allergies.

Skin Testing This is one of the most useful tests for physicians. Drops containing a potential allergen (e.g., house dust, pollen, mold, or another allergen) are placed on the back or forearm. The skin is pricked with a needle, allowing the allergen to enter the skin. This is called a prick test. A similar technique called a scratch test involves making a superficial scratch on the skin and dropping the allergen onto the scratch. In both

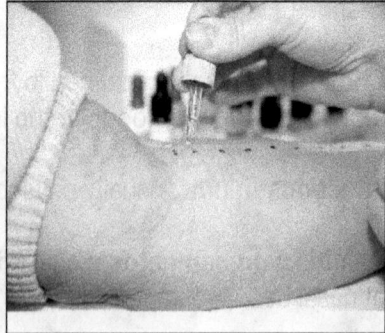

cases, an area of redness with swelling will develop if the person is allergic to the particular substance. The reaction usually occurs in about 15 minutes. If the reaction is severe, the allergen is wiped off the skin. The intensity of the reaction indicates how allergic one is to a substance. These results are used by the physician to confirm the diagnosis. It is possible to have a reaction to a certain allergen but not be clinically allergic to it; this means one may not have symptoms when exposed to the substance.

Blood Testing

Besides the skin testing, there is a second type of diagnostic testing for allergies, which is done on a blood sample.

You may wonder how blood can provide such accurate information about such a simple bodily activity as sneezing when you are exposed to pollen from the field next door. The answer lies in the body's highly developed immune system.

An allergic person "reacts abnormally" to pollen, dust, and so on, and creates more antibodies in the blood than somebody who is not allergic. (Antibodies are protein fighters that destroy or neutralize anything foreign that enters the body). If you look upon each allergen as a key – a ragweed key, a house dust key, a cat dander key, a birch tree key – you will see that they are all allergens, but each has a different shape or configuration.

The miracle of the body's defensive (immune) system is that the blood makes "locks" (antibodies) that can be matched to the "key" allergens. These are the IgE's we noted previously.

Laboratories can measure the amount of specific IgE antibody for each allergen present in the blood. This tells your physician exactly how much your body has "reacted abnormally" to each of the specific allergens, from the mold in your bathroom to the dust in your vacuum cleaner.

The most widely used and easy to perform blood testing system for the physicians' office is the ImmunoCAP provided by Phadia which is considered to be the most accurate and convenient for the patient. The picture shows how little blood is needed to measure your sensitivity to allergens.

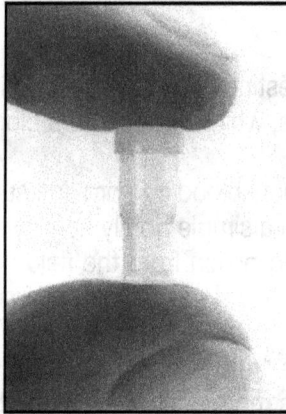

The reality is that hardly anybody is allergic to just one allergen. Therefore, a successful remedy depends on the ability to identify as many of your allergies as possible. This is especially true if the physician's treatment involves "allergy shots" (immunotherapy) or the avoidance of allergens in your environment.

COMPARISON OF BLOOD/SKIN TESTING

SKIN

Advantages

Immediate results (usually within 30 minutes).

It can be educational for the patient (demonstrating the allergic process of itching, swelling and redness.

It is relatively inexpensive.

Experienced physicians find the test sensitive in confirming suspected diagnosis.

Disadvantages

Not suitable for patients with a rash on forearm or back.

Not suitable for patients on antihistamine or some heart medications.

It can produce discomfort of itching, swelling and redness.

The process is time consuming, it can take 30 – 60 minutes.

There can a the risk of a severe allergic reaction (anaphylaxis).

BLOOD

Advantages

The test is not affected by taking medications such as antihistamines.

There is no possibility of a severe allergic reaction (anaphylaxis).

The process is quick (5 – 10 minutes)

The test can be done even if the patient has skin problems such as a rash.

It confirms definitively, yes or no if a patient is allergic to IgE mediated allergies.

Disadvantages

The test is more expensive.

The test result is not immediately available.

The test requires puncturing a vein to obtain a blood sample.

To qualify this comparison you must appreciate that both tests can be somewhat quantitative. The size of the skin test reaction relates to some extent the severity of the allergy. However the blood tests may be slightly more quantitative because the results are given in numbers.

However it is extremely important to note that a positive test does not always mean that the patient is allergic to the substance in question, and a negative test does not always mean that the patient is not allergic. Both tests have false-positive and false - negative results. In addition, both tests must be interpreted by a trained, experienced physician in order for their significance to be assessed.

In conclusion, it's important to understand that the accurate diagnosis of your allergic condition is very important for planning your most effective treatment plan. The only person who can do this is your physician, by reviewing not just the skin test or blood test, but your entire case history.

Specialists Who Can Help

☞ Physicians   ☞Allergy/immunologistspecialist

☞ Otolaryngologists   ☞ Primary Physicians

Other health care professionals that deal with Rhinitis:

☞ Pharmacists   ☞ Physician assistants

TREATMENT

Avoidance and Environmental Control

We have already pinpointed the most common causes or triggers of your symptoms, namely pollen(from grasses, weeds or trees), house dust mites, animal dander, molds or fungi, cockroaches, irritants, tobacco or wood smoke and viral respiratory infections.

Pollen is difficult to control when you are outside but you can control most of the other triggers to some extent. For more detailed specifics on planning your environmental control efforts we recommend two other books in this series: Allergy Avoidance in the Home and The Allergy Free Home.

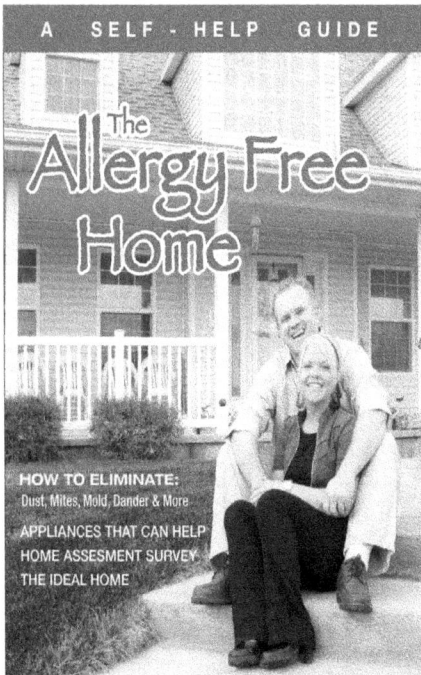

A SELF - HELP GUIDE

The Allergy Free Home

HOW TO ELIMINATE:
Dust, Mites, Mold, Dander & More
APPLIANCES THAT CAN HELP
HOME ASSESMENT SURVEY
THE IDEAL HOME

ENVIRONMENTAL CONTROL

The following tables provide information of reducing your exposure to the various allergens and irritants that can cause your rhinitis symptoms.

Check all the things that you think make your rhinitis symptoms worse

Allergens

Freshly mowed grass ☐
Dead grass ☐
Hay ☐
Dead leaves ☐
Pollen ☐
Trees/tree pollen ☐
Weeds (ragweed) ☐
Molds ☐
Cats/cat hair ☐
Dogs/dog hair ☐
Feathers ☐

Irritants

Smoke (tobacco/burning items) ☐
Perfumes/colognes/fragrances ☐
Cosmetics ☐
Cleaningproducts/detergents/soaps ☐
Paint fumes or paint products ☐
Hairspray ☐
outside dust ☐
Exhaust (cars, trucks, buses) ☐
Gasoline fumes ☐

Weather changes

Windy days ☐
Cold days ☐
Damp days ☐
Humidity/temperature changes ☐

Ingestants

Alcoholic beverages ☐
Spicy foods ☐

SOURCE	DESCRIPTION	POSSIBLE TRIGGER
Bedding	Old mattresses, pillows, box springs, duvets, blankets.	House dust mites, animal dander
Upholstered furniture	Old chairs, couches	House dust mites, animal dander
Appliances	Poorly maintained air conditioners, humidifiers, etc.	Mold
Poorly ventilated rooms	Rooms with no vents or windows especially in the laundry with no vent for the dryer or a crawl space	Mold, dust, dander
Clutter	Any type from ornaments, pictures, clothes or toys left around	Dust
Refrigerator	Especially those types with drip trays	Mold
Damp areas	Water damage, leaks, poorly ventilated bathroom	Mold, dust mites, cockroaches.
Food waste	Crumbs, food left on plates, garbage left unsealed	Cockroaches
Carpets	Old, decaying carpets, poorly cleaned	Dust mites, cockroaches
Drapes, curtains	Old and worn	Dust.
Pets	Any furry animal	Animal dander, dust
Air ducts	Without professional cleaning, can harbor triggers	Animal dander, dust, pollen
Garages	Cleaning materials, paints, chemical, in opened tins	Vapor irritants
Plants	Damp soil or unhealthy state	Mold/fungi
Home air quality	Air with a relative humidity of over 50% and warm temeperature	Dust mites, mold, cockroaches

ENVIRONMENTAL FACTOR	RECOMMENDATIONS FOR REDUCING EXPOSURE
Pollen	❏ Check out pollen counts on TV or in the newspaper so that you can be prepared. ❏ Avoid outdoor activities during periods of high pollen count. Usually they are highest early in the morning (dawn to 9.00AM) and in the early evening. ❏ Change clothes and shower after outdoor activities. ❏ Dry clothes in a vented area not outside in the open. ❏ Consider air conditioning and/or an air purifier in the bedroom. ❏ Keep windows and doors closed. ❏ Avoid using window or attic fans that draw air from the outside.
House dust mites	❏ Encase mattress, pillows and box springs within allergen barrier zippered covers. ❏ Wash bedding weekly in hot water (above 130° F). ❏ Reduce indoor humidity to 40%. ❏ Replace old carpets (especially in the bedroom). ❏ Try to substitute upholstered furniture with wood, leather or plastic furniture. ❏ Use a HEPA vacuum cleaner or central vacuum system. ❏ Wash stuffed toys in hot water and remove stuffed toys that cannot be washed or freeze them at least once weekly. ❏ Use acaricides (mitcides) as needed.
Mold/Fungi	❏ Reduce indoor humidity to less than 50% through air conditioning or a dehumidifier. ❏ Eliminate unnecessary dampness through water leaks or poor ventilation.

ENVIRONMENTAL FACTOR	RECOMMENDATIONS FOR REDUCING EXPOSURE
Mold/Fungi	❏ Clean at-risk surfaces with appropriate cleaner. ❏ Wash swamp coolers. ❏ For the outside, use the same tactics for pollen avoidance – also avoid areas such as uncut fields, raked leaves or areas with compost.
Animal dander	❏ Professionally clean the air ducts and close air ducts in the allergy sufferer's bedroom. ❏ Keep the pet out of the allergy sufferer's bedroom at all times. ❏ Keep the pet away from carpets and upholstered furniture. ❏ Apply dander controlling shampoos as recommended or wash the pet once a week. ❏ Remove the pet from the home.
Cockroaches	❏ Reduce food sources – clean up crumbs; wash dirty dishes and clean counters immediately; eat only in dining room or kitchen; don't leave pet's food out overnight; store food in tightly sealed containers; keep drawers, microwaves, ovens, and refrigerators clean and throw away or recycle grocery bags and newspapers. ❏ Reduce dampness – fix leaks; install a dehumidifier; remove rotted flooring or damp wallpaper; waterproof cement floors in garage and basement. ❏ Focus on at-risk areas – kitchen cabinets, floors and appliances; damp basements and bathrooms, toilets; anywhere there is food and water. ❏ Consider traps or an exterminator – for toxicity reasons, be careful setting traps if you have children; if your infestation is severe you may have to consider a professional exterminator.

ENVIRONMENTAL FACTOR	RECOMMENDATIONS FOR REDUCING EXPOSURE
Tobacco smoke	❏ Quit – it is difficult but there is help from your physician or pharmacist – there are medications and nicotine substitute products that can help dramatically. Talk to your pharmacist or physician and set a quit date. Second hand smoke affects everyone, not just allergy sufferers. ❏ Smoke outside – until you quit, you should smoke outside, certainly not in the home.
Wood smoke	❏ Ensure airtight stoves and fireplaces if wood must be burnt.
Viral upper respiratory infections	❏ Annual influenza shots – under the guidance of a health care professional these shots can reduce infection (these are contraindicated, however, for people who are sensitive to egg). ❏ Avoid contact with people with respiratory illnesses if possible. ❏ Wash hands frequently. ❏ Avoid sharing food, drinks and dishes.

MEDICATIONS

The objective of medication or pharmacotherapy is to alleviate and prevent a patient's allergy symptoms.

The medications used to treat allergic rhinitis are:

- Antihistamines
- Decongestants
- Antihistamine-decongestant combinations
- Corticosteroids
- Mast cell stabilizers
- Anticholinergics
- Leukotriene inhibitors

There are also some palliative treatments that can help such as:

- Nasal washes with warm salt water (with or without baking soda).
- Inhalation of warm mist through the nose for 10-15 minutes, 2 to 4 times a day, may also help.

Antihistamines are regarded as the first-line treatment for allergic rhinitis, and they are divided into two groups:

- Older, "first generation" compounds, also referred to as sedating antihistamines.

- Newer, "second generation" compounds, also referred to as non sedating or less sedating antihistamines.

How antihistamines work

Histamine is a chemical the body (specifically the mast cells and basuphils) releases in large quantities when reacting to an allergen. This chemical produces the symptoms of allergies; the antihistamines block the action and thereby relieve the nasal and eye symptoms of allergies.

A number of brands of these antihistamines can now be purchased at your pharmacy without a prescription.

There are substantial differences between these groups of antihistamines:

First generation antihistamines include such brand names as Benadryl® and Chlor-Tripolon®. These brands can cross the blood-brain barrier easily and can cause depressive reactions such as sedation, drowsiness and impairment in daily activities such as driving a car. These depressive side effects are not short-lived; even doses administered at bedtime may cause substantial sedation, decreased alertness, and impairment the following day. Another negative factor is that impairment or decreased cognitive ability that can occur in the absence of sedation and people may not be able to accurately determine how well they are performing tasks or even driving a car.

There are other related side effects such as dry mouth, constipations and urinary retention. These side effects are acknowledged as the most common and troublesome adverse effects and health care professionals usually discourage usage because of their high risk-to-benefit ratio.

Also, large doses of "first generation" antihistamines have the potential to induce life threatening or even fatal reactions.

Second generation antihistamines include such brand names as Claritin®, Zyrtec®, Alavert®, and Allegra®.

Many pharmacies have their own brand of the nonprescription antihistamines which can save money – you can check with your pharmacist on this issue.

These antihistamines have the major benefit of being non sedative or at least much decreased sedation. This is due to a lower tendency (unlike first generation antihistamines) to cross the blood-brain barrier. These drugs can be sedating, however, when the doses are exceeded.

Most of the second generation antihistamines have a fast onset of action (1 to 2 hours) and a long duration of action.

Unless there is some compelling reason to use a first generation antihistamine, you are probably choosing a "second generation" group of compounds.

Tips for optimizing antihistamine therapy

• Antihistamines are probably more effective given on a regular basis rather than 'as needed'- but clearly can be effective on an as needed basis as well, this is because most have a rapid onset of action.

• For predictable intermittent symptoms, the antihistamine should be administered daily during the period of allergen exposure.

- Exceeding the recommended dose of an antihistamine is unlikely to provide additional symptom relief.

- Exceeding the recommended dose of antihistamines can increase the incidence of adverse effects such as sedation.

- If patients do not experience adequate symptom relief from a second generation antihistamine, it is possible to obtain relief by switching to a different antihistamine. However, better results may be obtained by switching to an intranasal corticosteroid, or adding an intranasal corticosteroid to antihistamine therapy.

- Patient who understand the causes, symptoms and mechanisms of action of allergic rhinitis are more likely to comply to treatment and recommendations.

- Oral antihistamines generally are not effective against non-allergic symptoms. Treatment failure during antihistamine therapy could signal the presence of mixed rhinitis or pure non allergic rhinitis such as vasomotor rhinitis.

- All antihistamines should be discontinued several days before scheduled allergy skin tests because antihistamines decrease or prevent skin sensitivity.

Oral non-sedating antihistamines:

Generic Drug Name:	Trade Drug Name:	Adult Dosage:	Children Dosage:
Fexofenadine hydrochloride	Allegra™ Capsule	1 capsule (60 mg) twice daily Also available as 30mg & 180mg	12 yrs and older: same as adults
Loratidine	Claritin® Tablets	1 tablet (10 mg) once daily	12 yrs and older: same as adults
	Claritin® Reditabs	1 Reditab (10 mg once daily	12 yrs and older: same as adults
	Claritin® Syrup	2 tsp (5 mg/5 ml) once daily	2 through 5 yrs: 1 - 2 tsp once daily 6 through 11 years 1 - 2 tsp once daily
	Alavert®	1 (10mg) tablet daily	Age 2 to 6 yrs 5mg daily
Deslotradine	Clarinex®	5mg tablet. Physician decides dosage	Physician decides dosage
	Aerius® (Canada Only)		

Oral less-sedating antihistamines:

Generic Drug Name:	Trade Drug Name:	Adult Dosage:	Children Dosage:
Cetirizine hydrochloride	Zyrtec® Tablets	1-2 (5 mg) tablets once daily or 1 (10 mg) tablet once daily	12 yrs and older: same as adults 6 through 11 yrs: 1-2 tsp once daily
	Zyrtec® Syrup	1-2 tsp (5 mg/5 ml) once daily	2 through 5 yrs: start with ½ tsp once daily; may increase to 1 tsp once daily or ½ tsp twice daily

Intranasal antihistamines:

Generic Drug Name:	Trade Drug Name:	Adult Dosage:	Children Dosage:
Azelastine hydrochloride	Astelin® Nasal Spray	2 sprays (137mcg/spray) in each nostril 2 times a day	12 yrs and older: same as adults

37

Oral less-sedating antihistamines:

Generic Drug Name:	Trade Drug Name:	Adult Dosage:	Children Dosage:
Cetirizine hydrochloride	Zyrtec® Tablets	1-2 (5 mg) tablets once daily or 1 (10 mg) tablet once daily	12 yrs and older: same as adults 6 through 11 yrs: 1-2 tsp once daily
	Zyrtec® Syrup	1-2 tsp (5 mg/5 ml) once daily	2 through 5 yrs: start with ½ tsp once daily; may increase to 1 tsp once daily or ½ tsp twice daily
	Reactine® (Canada Only)		
Levecetirizine dihydrochloride	Xyzal® 5.0mg tablets	2.5mg (half tablet) - 5.0mg once daily in the evening	12 years or older 1-2 teaspoons or one tablet once daily in evening. 6-11 years old-1 teaspoon or half tablet once daily in evening
	Xyzal® Oral solutions	0.5mg/ml	12 years or older 1-2 teaspoons once daily in evening 6-11 years old 1 teaspoon once daily in evening

Intranasal antihistamines:

Generic Drug Name:	Trade Drug Name:	Adult Dosage:	Children Dosage:
Azelastine hydrochloride	Astelin® Nasal Spray	2 sprays (137mcg/spray) in each nostril 2 times a day	12 yrs and older: same as adults

Decongestants

How they work

Decongestants are known as sympathomimetic drugs because they affect the central nervous system and cause blood vessels to constrict. This reduces the supply of blood to the nose, decreases the amount the amount of blood in the sinuses, and decreases the mucosal swelling, which eventually improves nasal air flow.

These drugs primarily relieve the symptoms of nasal congestion or blockage. Although antihistamines are regarded as the first line treatment for allergic rhinitis, they are generally considered not as effective for alleviating nasal congestion symptoms. In fact, nasal congestion is sustained by a chronic inflammatory process and by numerous biochemicals other than histamine, which is why antihistamines have less effect on nasal congestion.

The most common decongestant available is phenylephrine and is available in either prescription or non prescription products, frequently in fixed dose combinations with antihistamines. Decongestants are available as oral or intranasal topical forms.
However, it is not advisable to take the nasal spray or topical products for more than 7 days because of side effects.

For this reason, there are several combination drugs available, combining antihistamines with decongestants to achieve a more comprehensive relief of nasal symptoms.

Oral decongestants

There can be several side effects of decongestants; these are dose dependant and related to the central nervous system (CNS) stimulation and systemic (all throughout the body) constriction of the blood vessels.

Possible CNS side effects include restlessness, insomnia, anxiety, tremors, fear and visual hallucinations. Vasoconstriction (blood vessel constriction) may cause elevated blood pressure, palpitations, tachycardia (fast heartbeat) and arrhythmias (abnormal rhythms of the heart). Oral decongestants should be used with caution.

Oral decongestants should not be used in pregnancy; they should also be avoided if you have diabetes, glaucoma, prostate enlargement or hyperthyroidism. They are also contraindicated in patients using monoamine oxidase inhibitors (MAO's) or patients who have received an MAO within the last two weeks.

Nose spray decongestants

Short courses of intranasal decongestants may be used to reduce severe nasal blockage which is beneficial in helping administer other needed intranasal medications such as corticosteroids. Intranasal decongestants are available as sprays or drops. They are categorized according to the duration of action.

• Short acting (4 to 6 hours): ephedrine, epinephrine, naphazoline, phenylephrine, and tetrahydrozoline
• Intermediate acting (8 to 10 hours): xylometazoline
• Long acting (greater than 10 hours): oxymetazoline

Intranasal decongestants work locally within the nose, so adverse effects generally are mild and infrequent.

Frequent use of these products, however, can cause a rebound effect of congestion known as rhinitis medicamentosa, so it is recommended to use intranasal decongestants for less than 5 days. The Drug Facts label for nonprescription products cautions patients to limit use to 3 days.

If rhinitis medicamentosa occurs, you should immediately discontinue taking nasal decongestants and either use nasal corticosteroids or start a short course of oral corticosteroids.

Antihistamine-decongestant combination medications

The previous section on antihistamines and decongestants will make you realize that these products may be more effective than either product used alone.

A further benefit may be that that the stimulatory effect of the decongestant may offset the sedating affect of the first generation antihistamines.

Oral non-sedating antihistamine-decongestant combinations

Generic Drug Name:	Trade Drug Name:	Adult Dosage:	Children Dosage:
Fexofenadine / Pseudoephedrine HCl	Allegra -D®	1 tablet (60mg) 2 times a day	12 yrs and older: same as adults
Loratadine / pseudoephedrine HCl	Claritin-D® 12 hour	1 tablet (5mg/120mg) 2 times daily	12 yrs and older: same as adults
	Claritin-D®	1 tablet (10mg/240mg) Once a day	12 yrs and older: same as adults

Oral less-sedating antihistamine-decongestant combinations

Generic Drug Name:	Trade Drug Name:	Adult Dosage:	Children Dosage:
Acrivastine/ pseudoephedrine HCl	Semprex - D® capsules	1 capsule (8mg/60mg), 4 times/day (every 4 -6 hours)	12 yrs and older: same as adults

Intranasal corticosteroids

How they work

These drugs are essentially anti-inflammatories; they help control inflammation and congestion by decreasing the swelling of the lining in the nasal passages and reducing nasal constrictions.

These are the most potent and efficacious medications currently available for the treatment of allergic rhinitis.

Nasal corticosteroids suppress many of the stages of the allergic inflammatory process and they are effective at improving all the usual symptoms of allergic rhinitis, including eye symptoms.

They are the preferred medication for adults with persistent symptoms of moderate to severe symptoms and are also often used in conjunction with antihistamines.

They are regarded as the first line of therapy when nasal obstruction is a major component of the rhinitis symptoms.

Intranasal corticosteroids are well tolerated; adverse effects are uncommon. Possible local adverse effects can include nasal irritation or burning sensation and nose bleed. The risk of these adverse effects can be minimized with proper administration techniques. You should direct the spray toward the outside of the nostril, away from the nasal septum. Holding the spray in the opposite hand can help facilitate the proper technique.

Intranasal corticosteroids are administered once daily, although twice daily administration may be necessary for severe symptoms and during flare ups of the symptoms.

Intra Nasal Corticosteroids

Generic Drug Name:	Trade Drug Name:	Adult Dosage:	Children Dosage:
Beclomethasone dipropionate	Beconase® Inhalation Aerosol	1 spray (42 mcg/spray) in each nostril 2-4 times/day	12 yrs and older: same as adults 6 to 12 yrs: 1 spray in each nostril 2-3 times/day
	Beconase AQ® Nasal Spray	1-2 sprays (42 mcg/ spray) in each nostril 2 times/day	12 yrs and older: same as adults 6 to 12 yrs: 1 spray in each nostril 2 times/day.
	Vancenase® Pockethaler Nasal Inhaler	1 spray (42 mcg/spray) in each nostril 2-4 times/day	12 yrs and older: same as adults 6 to 12 yrs: 1 spray in each nostril 2 times/day.
	Vancenase® AQ 84 mcg Nasal Spray	1-2 sprays (84 mcg/ spray) in each nostril 1 time/day	6 yrs and older: same as adults
Budesonide	Rhinocort® Nasal Inhaler	2 sprays (32 mcg/spray in each nostril twice daily or 4 sprays in each nostril each morning.	6 yrs and older: same as adults
Flunisolide	Nasarel® Nasal Solution	2 sprays (25 mcg/ spray) in each nostril twice daily; may increase to 2 sprays in each in each nostril 3-4 times/day (maximum 8 sprays in each nostril/day)	14 yrs and older: same as adults 6 to 14 yrs: 1 spray in each nostril 3 times/day or 2 sprays in each nostril twice daily (maximum 4 sprays in each nostril/day.
Fluticasone propionate	Flonase® Nasal Spray	2 sprays (50 mcg/spray) in each nostril once daily or 1 spray in each nostril twice daily.	4 yrs and older: same as adults, but start with 1 spray in each nostril once daily.

Intra Nasal Corticosteroids

Generic Drug Name:	Trade Drug Name:	Adult Dosage:	Children Dosage:
Mometasone furoate monohydrate	Nasonex® Nasal Spray	2 sprays (50 mcg/spray) in each nostril once daily	12 yrs and older: same as adults 3 to 12 yrs: 1 spray in each nostril once daily.
Triamcinolone	Nasacort® Nasal Inhaler	2 sprays (55 mcg/spray) in each nostril once daily; may increase to 2 sprays in each nostril twice daily or 1 spray in each nostril 4 times/day.	12 yrs and older: same as adults 6 through 11 years: 2 sprays in each nostril once daily.
	Nasacort® AQ Nasal Spray	2 sprays (55 mcg/spray) in each nostril once daily	12 yrs and older: same as adults 6 to 12 yrs: 1 spray in each nostril once daily; may increase to 2 sprays in each nostril once daily.
Fluticasone furoate	Veramyst	2 sprays (110mcg/spray in each nostril once daily	12 yrs and older: same as adults 2-11 years 1 spray in each nostril once daily

Cromolyn Sodium
(Mast cell stabilizer) (Nasalcrom®)

How it works

Intranasal cromolyn sodium is a topical over-the-counter non steroidal anti-inflammatory agent which has been described as a mast cell stabilizer; in fact, no one really knows how it works to relieve allergy rhinitis symptoms.

It is safe and well tolerated, but it is less effective than anti-histamines or intranasal corticosteroids.

The recommended frequency of dosage is 3 to 6 times daily, which could be inconvenient for patients and lead to poor treatment compliance.

It is used mostly as a preventative measure when a person knows they are going to be exposed to an allergen – for instance, when you visit a home that has a cat to which you are allergic. You have to continue therapy throughout the exposure period; it is not as effective when allergic symptoms have already started.

Intranasal mast cell stabilizers			
Generic Drug Name:	Trade Drug Name:	Adult Dosage:	Children Dosage:
Cromolyn Sodium	Nasalcrom®	1 spray (5.2 mg/spray) in each nostril 3 to 4 times/day (every 4 6 hours; may increase up to 6 times/day.	6 yrs and older: same as adults

Anticholinergic drugs
Ipratropium bromide (Atrovent®)

How it works

This medication is classified as an anticholinergic agent that inhibits nasal secretions by blocking certain receptors. It is available as a nasal spray and is effective in controlling watery nasal discharge, but it does not affect other symptoms of allergic rhinitis.

It is therefore not a first line treatment for allergic rhinitis for most patients. However, this medication may be useful by itself for a limited number of allergy sufferers who say their excessive runny noses (rhinorrhea) are their most troublesome side symptoms. It may be also used in combination with an antihistamine or intranasal corticosteroid for people whose rhinorrhea is not controlled well by other medications.

Intranasal Anticholinergics			
Generic Drug Name:	Trade Drug Name:	Adult Dosage:	Children Dosage:
Ipratropium bromide	Atrovent® Nasal spray 0.03% or 0.06%	2 sprays (21 mcg/spray) in each nostril 2-3 times/day.	6 yrs and older: same as adults 12 yrs and older: same as adults

Leukotriene receptor antagonists

How it works
They appear to be useful in calming nasal reactions.

Leukotriene receptor antagonists were first used to treat asthma. After several years of showing effectiveness in this disease, they were also approved for patients with rhinitis. They are therefore particularly useful for patients who have both diseases since there is a beneficial effect in both instances.

These medications appear to be comparable in effectiveness to oral antihistamines and less effective than intranasal corticosteroids. Some studies have shown that combination therapy with oral antihistamines provide additional benefits.

Leukotriene Modifiers			
Generic Drug Name:	Trade Drug Name:	Adult Dosage:	Children Dosage:
Montelukast	Singulair	10 mg tablets for 15 and older/one tablet in evening	5mg tablet chewable for ages 6 – 14 years old

The following chart shows how a specific drug type helps with the various allergy symptoms. It is of course always advisable to take the advice of an appropriate health care professional before changing medications.

This table represents a concensus of a medical task force's opinion. Referral with an appropriate health care professional is recommended

General Drug Management of Allergic Rhinitis		
DRUG	SNEEZING	ITCHING
Oral Antihistamines	Provides Substancial Benefits	Provides Substancial Benefits
Nasal Antihistamines	Provides Modest Benefit	Provides Modest Benefit
Intranasal Corticosteroids	Provides Substancial Benefits	Provides Substancial Benefits
Oral Decongestants	Provides No Benefit	Provides No Benefit
Intranasal Decongestants	Provides No Benefit	Provides No Benefit
Intranasal Mast cell stabilizers Chromolyn Sodium	Provides Modest Benefit	Provides Modest Benefit
Leuotriene receptor Antagonists	Provides No Benefit	Provides No Benefit
Topical Anticholinergics Ipatropium Bromide	Provides No Benefit	Provides No Benefit

General Drug Management of Allergic Rhinitis		
CONGESTION	RUNNY NOSE	EYE SYMPTOMS
Provides Little or Minimal Benefits	Provides Substancial Benefits	Provides Substancial Benefits
Provides Little or Minimal Benefits	Provides Modest Benefit	Provides No Benefit
Provides Substancial Benefits	Provides Substancial Benefits	Provides Modest Benefit
Provides Modest Benefit	Provides No Benefit	Provides No Benefit
Provides Substancial Benefits	Provides No Benefit	Provides No Benefit
Provides Modest Benefit	Provides Modest Benefit	Provides No Benefit
Provides Substancial Benefits	Provides Modest Benefit	Provides Substancial Benefits
Provides No Benefit	Provides Substancial Benefits	Provides Modest Benefit

TREATMENT APPROACHES

The professional recommendations for:

Seasonal allergic rhinitis

Commonly known as hayfever; usually associated with pollen from grasses, weeds and trees when they pollinate at various time of the year.

1. **Avoidance of pollen** - we cannot underestimate the importance of attempting to eliminate exposure to this trigger of rhinitis symptoms. Check out the relevant section in this book and seek further information.

2. **Anthihistamine usage** – this is the first-line medication option and is especially effective for the mild category of symptoms. Antihistamines reduce the symptoms of runny nose, itching and sneezing and can reduce the symptoms of watery eyes (allergic conjunctivitis). However, they have little effect on nasal congestion or post nasal drip (that uncomfortable feeling at the back of the throat).

   There are various brands which fall into two categories: first generation such as Benadryl®, Chlorotriptono ®, and Dimetapp®, and second generation such as Claritin®, Allergra®, Zyrtec®, Alavert®, Reactine® (in Canada) and many generic brands in pharmacies.

3. **Nasal decongestant** – these are a type of precision medications used to relieve nasal congestion and/or post nasal drip. These products are available as a spray (which is more rapid in relieving symptoms) or as an oral medication. However, using the topical application for more than a week can bring on a side effect called rhinitis medicamentosa.

4. **Antihistamine and decongestant usage** – as antihistamines do not solve the problem of nasal congestion and post nasal drip, taking a combination of therapy of these two dugs is quite common. There are various brands such as Allegra-D®, Claritin-D® (12 hour and 24 hour) and Semprex-D®.

5. **Corticosteroids** – these are potent drugs for seasonal allergic rhinitis, usually used as a nasal spray. They are very useful when nasal obstruction or blockage is a troubling component of the symptoms. They have a less rapid action than the antihistamines so they should be taken regularly for best results.

The nasal spray is broken down quickly in the nasal membranes so there is very little worry about systemic or body side effects. Some brands include: Beconase®, Vancenase®, Rhinocort®, Nasarel®, Flonase®, Nasonex® and Nasacort®.

Oral corticosteroids have a quicker onset of action to relieve symptoms but they should be only used for 3 to 7 days because of potential side effects.

6. **Cromolyn Sodium** – for maximum effect it should be administered prophylactically before exposure to the allergen, e.g. before mowing the grass. Side effects are minimal and it is safe for children and pregnant women. It does have to be administered 4 to 6 times daily.

Perennial (all year round) allergic rhinitis

Unlike seasonal allergens, animal dander, dust mites, and mold are present in the home environment all year long, usually leading to persistent symptoms.

1. **Allergen avoidance** – you should not underestimate this aspect of treatment; there are more ways to avoid allergens in the home than in the outdoors. See the previous section on allergen avoidance and review the other books in this series Allergy Avoidance in the Home and The Allergy Free Home.

2. **Topical (nasal spray)corticosteroids** – these are usually preferred for the chronic (unremitting) symptoms of this condition. This is especially true when nasal congestion is a predominant, troubling symptom.

3. **Other medications** – antihistamines, antihistamine-decongestant combinations and Chromolyn Sodium can also be used in the right circumstances.

Chronic non-allergic rhinitis (Vasomotor rhinitis)

This is a difficult type of rhinitis to treat; avoidance of the irritant is often difficult to achieve, either because of a person's heightened sensitivity to these irritants or because the person simply does not know which irritant to avoid. The two most common treatments are:

Nasal spray antihistamine: Astelin® has shown to be very effective in both allergic and non-allergic rhinitis; a response rate of 82- 85% for vasomotor rhinitis has been reported. Astelin® seems to relieve most of the rhinitis symptoms including nasal congestion, runny nose, postnasal drainage and sneezing.

Topical (nasal spray) corticosteroids – these are potent drugs which should be taken regularly to alleviate the symptoms and because they are metabolized. Two corticosteroids have been approved for non allergic rhinitis: Fluticasone® and Beclomethasone®.

Decongestants – these are recommended for the specific symptom of nasal congestion or obstruction with non allergic rhinitis if other treatments have failed. Again, nasal sprays should be used for no longer than 7 days and only oral decongestants should be used for the long term.

Anticholinergic (Atrovent®) – this is the first line treatment nasal spray for vasomotor rhinitis where the predominant symptom is excessive runny nose (rhinorrhea). Sometimes it is preferable to use this product in conjunction with a topical corticosteroid; the two combined drugs have an additive effect compared with the use of either drug alone.

Mixed rhinitis

This is the term for when a patient has allergic rhinitis whose symptoms are clearly worsened by non-allergic triggers such as strong odors, weather conditions, fumes or cigarette smoke. This diagnosis is based upon the physician's interpretation of all the factors.

Astelin® - this is the only intranasal antihistamine indicated for mixed rhinitis; it is a reasonable first choice because of its broad based nature and is fairly comprehensive in relieving nasal symptoms.

Other specific medications – can be chosen to target specific symptoms if they are not being controlled. Decongestants, anticholinergics and palliative saline and topical nasal steroids can be useful additions when appropriate.

Cholinergic rhinitis

This describes the copious rhinorrhea (runny nose) triggered by spicy foods or the inhalation of cold, dry air that often occurs with skiers and joggers.

Atrovent® (Ipratropium Bromide) – this first line of treatment is taken prophylactically, usually two sprays in each nostril 45 to 60 minutes before eating or exposure to cold air.

Occupational rhinitis

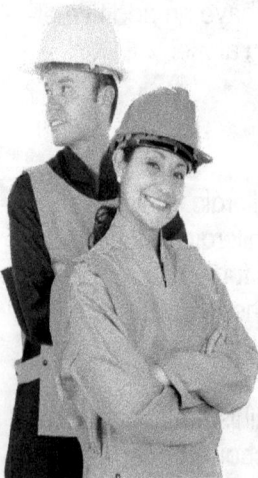

This is allergic or non-allergic rhinitis developed by exposure at work.

Avoidance – this is the mainstay of treatment by removing the allergen or irritant, improving ventilation, wearing a mask or even changing the work site.

Saline wash – a nasal saline wash can help by removing the accumulated particles from the nose area.

SPECIAL CATEGORIES OF ALLERGY SUFFERERS

PREGNANT WOMEN

Safety is the major principle guiding the choice of medication for pregnant women. If you are pregnant, try steam inhalation, saline nasal sprays and avoidance of the allergens or irritants before considering using medication.

The development of rhinitis in pregnancy could be hormonal driven – body changes can exacerbate a previously existing mild rhinitis by increasing nasal congestion. There is a massive expansion of circulating blood volume during pregnancy which in turn can increase nasal "pooling" of the blood, contributing to the rhinitis symptoms. Nasal congestion is common during the second half of the pregnancy

As a general rule for treating pregnant women with rhinitis, topical treatments (nasal sprays) are preferred.

Chromolyn Sodium is one of the safest medications to use and is considered the first choice.

If this does not work or is not practical then **nasal spray corticosteroids** should be considered.

Claritin®, Zyrtec®, Montelukask and Rhinocorv AQ can be used to treat Rhinitis in pregnancy.

In the third trimester, the decongestant **pseudoephedrine** may be considered to treat the nasal congestion specifically.

Antihistamines may be considered under certain circumstance under the guidance of a health care professional.

Always consult with your physician concerning any medication you may take during pregnancy.

ELDERLY PATIENTS

The same medication guidelines apply to the elderly as have been described in the medication section of this book. There are, however, some cautionary considerations to be aware of in the management of rhinitis in the elderly.

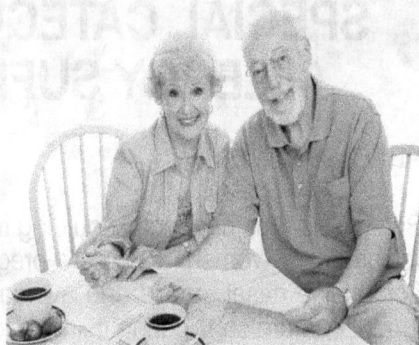

Allergy is a less common cause of both perennial and seasonal rhinitis in individuals over 65 years of age. Atrophy (shrinkage and aging of nasal tissue) can be the cause of this difficult-to-treat condition in older individuals.

You should consider drug induced rhinitis as a possible diagnosis especially if the patient is using any of these medications: Reserpins®, Guanethidine®, Phentolamine®, Methyldopa®, Prazosin®, Chlorpromazine® or ACE inhibitors.

As mentioned previously decongestants may cause urinary retention and cardiac and CNS (central nervous system) stimulation may be a concern.

Selecting the appropriate antihistamine is important because the side effect of sedation, especially with the first generation antihistamines, may contribute to falling and subsequent injury, such as a fracture. In some patients bladder disturbances or visual problems may occur with antihistamines.

CHILDREN

The same guidelines can be applied for children from the medication section, with the recommended reduced dosages. There are some qualifying factors that should be appreciated in the treatment and diagnosis issues.

Often the diagnosis of allergic rhinitis can be missed in children due to the symptoms of otitis media (ear infection) and other ear, nose and throat conditions. Although one should keep an open mind when diagnosing a child's symptoms, it is known that allergic rhinitis is unusual in children under 3 years of age.

Allergy tests such as skin or blood tests can be performed on children at any age and may yield important information. In fact, early recognition of allergic rhinitis can lead to reduced complications. Once a trigger has been identified and you are trying to take avoidance measures in the home, it is important to evaluate the potential exposure of the same allergen at the school or day care premises.

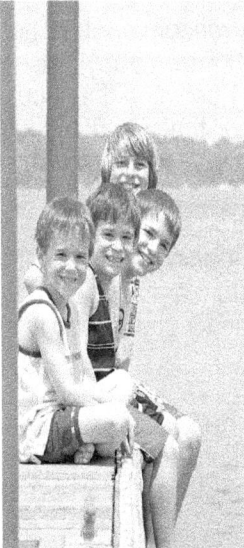

There is evidence that the symptoms of allergic rhinitis can impair school performance; this can be made worse if children are using the sedating antihistamines.

IMMUNOTHERAPY (ALLERGY SHOTS)

This treatment is a series of injections (shots) with a solution containing the allergen that causes your symptoms. Treatment usually begins with a weak solution given once or twice a week. The strength of the solution is gradually increased with each dose. Once the strongest dose is reached, the injections are often given once a month to ensure control of your symptoms.

It may take 6 months to a year before you notice any improvement in symptom reduction.

In theory you have decreased your sensitivity, or desensitized yourself, to the allergen and have now reached your maintenance level, requring less frequent injections. This is similar to the concept of being vaccinated against viruses.

The process

The injections are usually only slightly uncomfortable, not painful, and are normally given in the loose (floppy) tissue over the back of the upper arm, halfway between the shoulder and elbow – this is under the skin or the subcutaneous tissue. Small diabetic insulin syringes are used to inject the allergens.

It is important to appreciate that you are being injected with a commercially extracted allergen with standardized potency. Nobody has obtained house dust from under your couch and put it into a syringe!

You should always be injected in the physician's office and wait there for 30 minutes after the injection, just in case you have a serious reaction. If that happens, trained personnel will be available to treat you immediately.

How it works

Allergy shots alter the way your immune system reacts to an allergen. By giving small but increasing amounts of the allergen at regular intervals, tolerance to the allergen increases. The end result is that you can become immune to the allergens and tolerate them with fewer symptoms.

Who is suitable for allergy immunotherapy?

1. People with seasonal allergic rhinitis or allergic asthma where:
    a) It is difficult or impossible to successfully avoid the cause
    b) Medication does not seem to work
    c) Medication causes side effects
    d) As an alternative to medication

2. People with perennial (all year round) allergic rhinitis where there is a significant progression of symptoms that is dramatically affecting their quality of life.

3. People who have dangerous allergic reactions (anaphylaxis) to stinging insects like bees, wasps or fire ants.
The following conditions must apply:

a) That there is appropriate standardized potent extracts (for the injection) available to implement the immunotherapy program, and

b) There is clear evidence of a relationship between symptoms and exposure to an unavoidable allergen to which the patient is sensitive.

What is the success rate?

In stinging insect allergies (bee, wasp, hornets, yellow jackets and so on), the protection against dangerous severe allergic reactions (anaphylaxis) is quoted at 80 to 95%.

Three out of four patients with seasonal allergic reactions experience significant improvement with immunotherapy. However, sometimes symptoms are reduced rather than abolished and some medication may still be needed.

Well controlled clinical studies have demonstrated that immunotherapy is beneficial in the treatment of allergic rhinitis caused by:

- Tree pollens
- Grass pollens
- Weed pollens
- Mold spores
- Dust mites
- Animal dander

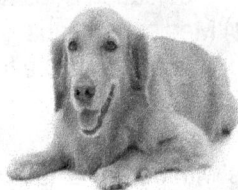

Some controlled studies have shown allergen immunotherapy provides significant clinical improvement based on reduced symptom scores (medication use, office visits, unscheduled office visits and improved pulmonary function tests) for patients with:
Seasonal pollen – and mold – induced asthma
Perennial (all year round) allergic asthma caused by animal dander and dust mites.

PATIENT PROFILES

David T. operates a fork-lift truck for a magazine distribution company. He always gets a runny nose, itching, sneezing and watery eyes during the ragweed pollen season. David says he can live with it, most of the time, but it does affect his quality of life at the height of the pollen season, when the symptoms get much worse.

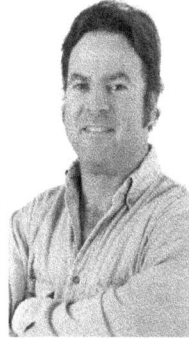

Treatment: David's case is relatively mild and seasonal, so oral antihistamines from his physician are appropriate treatment – in David's case, his pharmacist supplied him with a generic brand. It was critical for him to use the second generation antihistamines; the product his pharmacist recommended is a pharmacy chain's generic equivalent of Claritin. It has no sedating effects so David can still do his job.

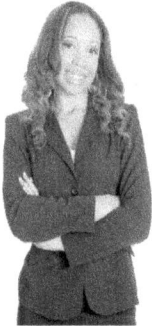

Eleanor W. a marketing administrator for an insurance company, has developed an allergy to cat dander. In fact, she had to give her beloved pet Siamese to a relative because of her condition. Tonight, she is going to dinner at a friend's house. The friend has two cats and Eleanor fears she may have an allergy attack.

Treatment: Eleanor can simply take an oral antihistamine before setting off for her friend's house or even when she arrives, because antihistamines are fast-acting. Alternatively, she can take Cromolyn Sodium prophylactically because this is an isolated exposure and she can plan for it.

Sylvie L. the mother of two teenage boys, teaches design part-time at a local college. She is a classic multi-sensitive allergic patient with allergies to house dust mites, mold, cats and dogs, causing severe nasal congestion. If she does not take her medication, Sylvie experiences chronic debilitating symptoms all year long.

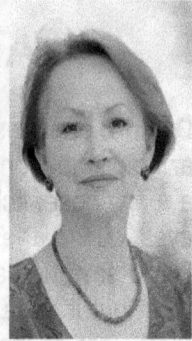

Treatment: Sylvie's physician prescribed a nasal spray corticosteroid a few years ago and she takes it every day to prevent symptoms occurring. Previously, she had taken non-prescription, first generation antihistamines; these worked fine but the sedating side effects were a problem. Occasionally, when she feels it's necessary, Sylvie will use a second generation antihistamine as a booster, and sometimes she'll use a combination antihistamine with decongestant when the nasal decongestion seems to be developing.

Brian A. is a technologist at a hospital. His problem is that, even after several tests, his physician cannot pinpoint all of his triggers or allergens. Brian seems to have mixed rhinitis made much worse by soaps, perfumes, and all kinds of fumes. His symptoms include nasal congestion, watery eyes, sneezing and itching.

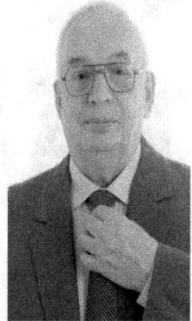

Treatment: Brian's physician prescribed a broad based, non-specific therapy, Astelin, which is the only available antihistamine nasal spray. This has proven to be effective for both allergic and non-allergic rhinitis and, equally important, it is usually effective with all the allergy nasal symptoms including nasal congestion.

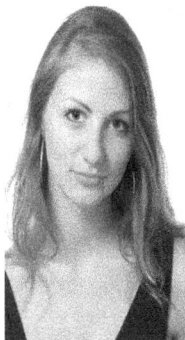

Brenda T. works in the accounting department of a paper mill and seems extremely sensitive to a wide range of irritants, from tobacco smoke and hairspray to food odors. Her physician has classified her allergy as vasomotor rhinitis. The main symptomatic problem for Brenda is a copious runny nose (rhinorrhea) which she finds very embarrassing, especially at work.

Treatment: Brenda's physician prescribed the only anticholinergic drug available, Atrovent®, which is very effective at eliminating the excessive runny nose symptom. In fact, a stronger formulation is used by physicians to prevent runny noses for patients suffering from a bad cold. For some patients, although not in Brenda's case, topical corticosteroids can be used as well to ensure complete suppression of the symptoms.

Brenda also finds she gets relief by administering nasal saline washes. Commercial brands are available at the pharmacy which can provide symptomatic relief.

SELF-TREATING
AT THE PHARMACY

As a patient, you may seek non prescription medications for relief of allergy symptoms, for one of any of the following reasons:

a. You have already been diagnosed as having allergic rhinitis.
b. You want to save costs
c. Your health care practitioner may have recommended you to go to the pharmacist for allergy relief medication
d. You may have made a correct diagnosis of suffering from allergy symptoms and are seeking quick relief.
e. You may have a common cold, a viral infection or asthma and think it is allergy, so you consider a trip to the pharmacy is in order.

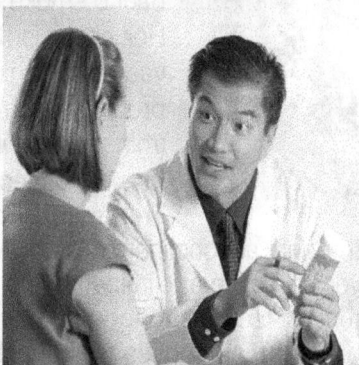

In any of these cases you should ensure you discuss fully with the pharmacy staff your motivations and symptoms to ensure a healthy outcome. They are there to help you and are well-qualified to do so.

In most cases, your pharmacist will recommend a type of antihistamine. It is important, however, for your pharmacist to have some key questions answered beforehand.

Here is a list of questions for which your pharmacists needs answers:

Patient Questionnaire

1. In the past 12 months, how many times have the symptoms occurred?

☐ Less than 4 days a week or less than 4 weeks in a year?

☐ More than 4 days a week and more than 4 weeks in a year?

2. In the past 12 months have these nose disturbances been accompanied by sleep disturbance?

☐ Yes
☐ No

3. In the past 12 months, how much have these nose problems interfered with you?
A (not at all) B (a little) C (a moderate amount) D (a lot)

	A	B	C	D
Daily activities	☐	☐	☐	☐
School	☐	☐	☐	☐
Work	☐	☐	☐	☐
Leisure	☐	☐	☐	☐
Sport	☐	☐	☐	☐

DETERMINING THE SEVERITY OF ALLERGY

A new classification of allergic rhinitis has been developed by an authoritative group called the ARIA (Allergic Rhinitis and the impact on Asthma) to address the shortcomings and dynamically fluctuating nature of \patient symptoms due to having both seasonal and perennial rhinitis etc.

To keep matter simple the ARIA have categorized allergic rhinitis as either intermittent or persistent, depending on the severity of the symptoms (see following chart). These categories of patients are graded according to the severity of either mild or moderate - severe based upon the presence or absence of four health related quality of life items as shown in box D.

Consequently patients may be categorized into one of four categories of allergic rhinitis:

mild intermittent
moderate severe intermittent
Mild persistent
Moderate - severe

Interpreting the severity of your allergies
If you reported the presence of one, two or three items in box D, you would be classified as having moderate allergies; patients who reported ALL FOUR items in Box D would be classified as having severe allergies.
If you ticked Box A then you have **intermittent** symptoms
If you ticked Box B then you have **persistent** symptoms
If you ticked all of the boxes in Box C you have **mild** symptoms

BOX A

Intermittent Symptoms

☐ Less than 4 days a week
☐ Less than 4 weeks a year

BOX B

Persistent Symptoms

☐ More than 4 days a week
☐ More than 4 weeks a year

BOX C

Mild

☐ All of the following
☐ Normal sleep
☐ No impairment of daily activities, sports, leisure
☐ No impairment of work or school
☐ No troublesome symptoms

BOX D

Moderate - Severe

☐ One or more items
☐ Abnormal sleep
☐ Impairment of daily activities, sports, leisure
☐ Impaired work and school
☐ Troublesome symptoms

The conclusions or rule of thumb for a course of action are as follows.

• People who report only **intermittent or mild symptoms** (Box A & C) can self treat successfully with a nonprescription second generation antihistamine (or an antihistamine/decongestant product).

• People who report **moderate to severe intermittent** symptoms (Box A & D) may attempt self treatment; however they should consult a physician if no improvement is noted within 7 to 15 days of therapy.

- People who report **moderate to severe AND persistent** symptoms (boxes B & and D)   should be evaluated by a physician rather than rely on self treatment. (These patients are likely to obtain better symptom control with intranasal corticosteroids).

As a footnote to this clever way of categorizing allergies; it is meant to be a fluid system in which patients move among the categories depending upon the allergies getting worse or you are controlling your allergies. For example, a patient may have mild but persistent symptoms of allergic rhinitis for most of the year. However with the advent of the ragweed pollen season in the Summer the symptoms can progress to moderate - severe.

In fact this is seen in clinical practice where a major proportion of patients visit their primary care provider when their symptoms are categorized as moderate - severe. This may demonstrate the tendency for patients to visit their health care provider only when they are significantly troubled by the allergy symptoms.

If this is your case, you may want to consider being treated for your mild symptoms throughout the year on the occasions that may just affect your quality of life. You may then be more prepared with an understanding of how to use your medications, when moderate - severe symptoms occur.

There are very definite exclusions for self-treatment of allergic rhinitis which your pharmacy will know but it is worth highlighting these factors:

Exclusions for self-treatment of allergic rhinitis

• Children younger than 12 years of age

• Pregnant women or women who are breastfeeding

• Symptoms not associated with allergic rhinitis (already listed)

• Severe persistent allergic rhinitis

• Symptoms of undiagnosed asthma

• Symptoms of uncontrolled asthma

• Ear ache

• Symptoms unresponsive to treatment

• Unacceptable adverse effects of treatment

CONCLUSION

This book has been an attempt to translate the health care professional's best practice guidelines and information on allergic and non allergic rhinitis into an easy to understand format.

The subject of allergies is wide and it must be emphasized that this book mostly focuses upon the allergies that account for most of the problems. There are many other types of allergies such as food allergies or allergic conjunctivitis of the eye that are from a symptom standpoint as equally as troubling for the patient as the allergies discussed in this book.

Furthermore, there are other causes of allergies that we have not discussed such as latex allergies or allergies to specific drugs such as penicillin. Technically you can almost be allergic to anything.

Here are some of the conditions with an allergic component that we did either did not cover in this book or did not discuss in any detail. You may find more information on the Internet, by talking to your doctor or in other books in this series:

Conjunctivitis: this refers to a group of inflammation type eye disorders.

Urticaria and Angioderma: skin disorders.

Contact dermatitis: skin reaction due to skin contact with a substance from either the work place or anywhere else.

Drug reactions: are reactions to a drug or biological agent. It is estimated that 10% of all drug reactions are due to allergic reactions.

Insect sting reactions: This can cause the most severe of all allergic reactions leading to death.

Food allergies: is a group of disorders, the most serious being anaphylaxis as in the insect sting category. The prevalence of food allergies is greatest in the first few years of life.

Latex reactions: this is caused by the protein in latex in gloves, balloons, condoms etc. This type of allergy is increasing and is of special concern to health care professionals.

Anaphylaxis: this is life threatening allergic reactions, common in some food and insect sting allergies. It is important to be knowledgeable on this topic because of the consequences.

Our goal is to help you to understand what allergies are and how they are caused and introduce basic information around treatment options, the most important of which is to avoid the allergen altogether, if you can.

We have listed a range of medication options together with a comparative review linked to symptoms and have explained the newest and most practical approach to classifying the symptoms - ARIA (Allergy Rhinitis and the Impact on Asthma) - with its linkage to appropriate treatment. This is especially important because so many patients self treat and medication decisions can be made between pharmacist and patient. It is always advisable to have as much information that is available to make the right joint decisions.

There is no cure for allergies, although in some patients they may go away naturally. The main issue (apart from the life threatening anaphylaxis) is one's quality of life, which is linked to symptom relief.

The loss of productivity at work or at school and the impairment of social functions due to allergies have been well documented. The positive news is that avoidance, medications or allergy shots can effectively control allergy symptoms. Used on a daily basis, as recommended by your doctor or pharmacist, these medications are quite safe.

Many thousands of people suffer from allergies and are not benefiting from the available treatment. This is a diagnosis issue; as a patient or caregiver, you need to be proactive and seek help from your pharmacist or health care professional. Only when you truly know "the enemy" will you stand a chance of beating the runny nose, sneezing, watery eyes and all of the other debilitating symptoms affecting your quality of life.

USEFUL INFORMATION WEBSITES

Internet directory of allergy organizations and resources
www.allallergy.net

Allergy and Asthma Foundation of America (AAFA)
www.aafa.org

Allergy and Asthma Network Mothers of Asthmatics (AAN/MA)
www.aanma.org

American Academy of Allergy, Asthma and Immunology (AAAAI)
www.aaaai.org

American College of Allergy, Asthma and Immunology (ACAAI)
www.allergy.mcg.edu

American Lung Association
www.lungusa.org

Allergy and Asthma Information
www.allergyasthmaclient.com

National Air Duct Cleaners Association (NADCA)
www.nadca.com

Pollen Counts
www.pollen.com

Health House information - Lung Association
www.healthyhouse.org

Footnotes

American Academy of Allergy, Asthma, and Immunology website. Retrieved March 26, 2008 from http://www.aaaai.org/media/resources/media_kit/allergy_statistics.stm.

Schoenwetter, W. F., L. Dupclay, Jr., S. Appajosyula, et al. Economic impact and quality-of-life burden of allergic rhinitis. Curr Med Res Opin. 2004; 20:305-317.

Kay, G. G. The effects of antihistamines on cognition and performance. J Allergy Clin Immunol. 2000; 105(suppl):S622-27.

Blaiss, M. S. Allergic rhinoconjunctivitis: burden of disease. Allergy Asthma Proc. 2007; 28:393-397.

Goetzel, R. Z., S. R. Long, R. J. Ozminkowski, et al. Health, absence, disability, and presenteeism cost estimates of certain physical and mental health conditions affecting U. S. employers. J Occup Environ Med. 2004; 46:398-412.

Reed, S. D., T. A. Lee & D. C. McCrory. The economic burden of allergic rhinitis. Pharmacoeconomics. 2004; 22:345-361.

American Academy of Allergy, Asthma and Immunology website.

Leger, D., I. Annesi-Maesano, F. Carat, et al. Allergic rhinitis and its consequences on quality of sleep: an unexplored area. Arch Intern Med. 2006; 166:1744-1748.

Adkinson, N. F. Jr., J. W. Yunginger, W. W. Busse, et al., eds., Middleton's Allergy: Principles and Practice. 6th ed. Philadelphia, PA: Mosby; 2003.

Bousquet, J., P. van Cauwenberge, N. Khaltaev, et al. ARIA in the pharmacy: management of allergic rhinitis symptoms in the pharmacy. Allergy. 2004; 59:373-387.

G. S. Rachelefsky. National guidelines needed to manage rhinitis and prevent complications. Ann Allergy Asthma Immunol. 1999; 82:296-305.

Bousquet, et al.

Adkinson, et al.

Lehman, J. M. & M. S. Blaiss. Selecting the optimal oral antihistamine for patients with allergic rhinitis. Drugs. 2006; 66:2309-2319.

Bousquet, J., et al. 2001.

American Academy of Allergy, Asthma, and Immunology website. Tips to Remember: What is Allergy Testing? Retrieved March 27, 2008 from http://www.aaaai.org/patients/publicedmat/tips/whatisallergytesting.stm.

Bousquet, J., et al. 2001.

Adkinson, N. F. Jr.

Bousquet, J., et al. 2001.

Bousquet, J., et al. 2004.

Bousquet, J., et al. 2001.